One Word ENCOURAGE Journal

One Word ENCOURAGE Journal

MARY P. WELLS

Contents

Dedication

To my son, Kaleb, the reason I keep going. It is an honor to be "Mom." Thank you for being by my side and sharing God's Word. Your precious smile brightens my spirit.

To those who undergo cancer, this journal is written to remind you to speak, reflect and write encouraging words in the midst of your journey. If you are unable to do so, your Support Team Member can journal as he/she cheers you on to the finish line victorious! During your quiet moments rejoice in knowing that each day is a gift that you live!

Introduction

In this world, everyone encounters challenges. We are not exempt from them. The question is, "How to face challenges that come out of nowhere?" The answer is in the way we respond. Take captive of your challenges by identifying they exist and speaking the outcome.

This journal is written for the purpose to read God's encouraging Words and to speak positively to your challenges. While fighting breast cancer, I recall the side effects of chemotherapy were so severe that I was unable to write in my journal midway through treatment. As I look back, I think about what could have been written if I asked a Support Team Member to continue journaling for me. My Support Team spoke encouraging words into me when I did not for myself. I appreciate their persistence because I began to speak encouraging words. What we say shapes our lives.

Today, I continue to speak encouraging words, not only in all areas of my life but also in people all over the world. I am six years cancer-free and healed! You can declare freedom and healing from your challenges by consistently speaking encouraging words over every area of your life.

A is for ABLE

Now until Him who is able to do immeasurably more than all we ask or imagine, according to his power that is at work within us. — Ephesians 3:20 (NIV)

- God is able to do more than you can imagine;
- God's power is working within you;
- You are able to do anything. Draw from the power of God within you to do it!

I am **ABLE** to do:

_____

_____

_____

_____

_____

_____

_____

_____

_____

_____

_____

B is for BURIED

For we died and we were buried with Christ by baptism. —
Romans 6:4a (NLT)

- Your past is not brought into the present or future;
- Your sins are forgiven, erased;
- At baptism, your past is buried and no longer exists.

What I BURY:

_____

_____

_____

_____

_____

_____

_____

_____

_____

_____

_____

C is for CREATED

So God created human beings in his own image. In the image
God he created them; male and female he created them. —
Genesis 1:27 (NLT)

- God created you;
- The way you are created is how God imagined;
- You are wonderfully created.

As I look in the mirror, I am **CREATED**:

_____

_____

_____

_____

_____

_____

_____

_____

_____

_____

D is for DELIVERED

You are my hiding place; you will protect me from trouble and surround me with songs of deliverance. — Psalm 32:7 (NIV)

- God hides you when in trouble;
- God is your protection;
- Trouble no longer exists because God delivers you.

I am **DELIVERED** from:

_____

_____

_____

_____

_____

_____

_____

_____

_____

_____

_____

E is for ETERNAL

*And this what God has testified: He has given us eternal life,
and this life is in his Son. — 1 John 5:11 (NLT)*

- Life in the world is temporary;
- You have eternal life given by God;
- Eternal life is only in God's Son, Jesus Christ.

My **ETERNAL** life is:

_____

_____

_____

_____

_____

_____

_____

_____

_____

_____

_____

_____

F is for FORGIVE

And forgive us our sins, as we have forgiven those who sin against us. — Matthew 6:12 (NLT)

- When praying, ask God to forgive your sins;
- When praying, forgive others who sin against you;
- Asking God for forgiveness & forgiving others go hand in hand.

God **FORGIVE** me:

G is for GIVE

Give us today the food we need. — Matthew 6:11 (NLT)

- When you pray, acknowledge God is provider;
- God provides food for today;
- Your needs are met.

God **GIVE** me today:

_____

_____

_____

_____

_____

_____

_____

_____

_____

_____

_____

_____

H is for HELP

My help comes from the Lord, the Maker of heaven and earth.
— Psalm 121: 2 (NIV)

- Your help comes from the Lord;
- There's only one Lord who made heaven and earth;
- Go to the Lord for help.

Lord **HELP** me:

I is for INCREASE

A wise man has great power, and a man of knowledge increases strength. — Proverbs 24:5 (NIV)

- Your knowledge is from God;
- Your strength is from God;
- Wisdom is a vital part of strength.

As I I**NCREASE** God's knowledge in my life, I have strength to do the following:

_____

_____

_____

_____

_____

_____

_____

_____

_____

_____

_____

J is for JOY

Consider it pure joy, my brothers and sisters, whenever you face trials of many kinds. — James 1:2 (NIV)

- Trials continue throughout your life;
- Trials are temporary;
- Remain joyous because you are an overcomer.

I have **JOY** during this trial(s):

_____

_____

_____

_____

_____

_____

_____

_____

_____

_____

_____

_____

_____

K is for KEEP

The Lord will keep you from all harm – He will watch over your life. — Psalm 121:7 (NIV)

- The Lord keeps you from current and future harm;
- The Lord is your protector;
- The Lord always watches over you.

God **KEEPS** me from:

_____

_____

_____

_____

_____

_____

_____

_____

_____

_____

_____

_____

L is for LOVE

Love never fails. — *1 Corinthians 13:8a (NIV)*

- Love always;
- Love is what you give to everyone;
- Love is the greatest.

I am to **LOVE**:

_____

_____

_____

_____

_____

_____

_____

_____

_____

_____

_____

M is for MADE

I praise you because I am fearfully and wonderfully made.
— Psalm 139: 14 (NIV)

- Thank God for how you are made;
- God made you fearfully;
- God made you wonderfully.

God has **MADE** me:

_____

_____

_____

_____

_____

_____

_____

_____

_____

_____

N is for NEW

For I am about to do something new. See, I have already begun! Do you not see it? I will make a pathway through the wilderness. I will create rivers in the dry wasteland. — Isaiah 43:19 (NLT)

- You are a new person;
- You are living a new life created by God;
- God makes your paths that were once dead now alive.

My **NEW** Life is:

_____

_____

_____

_____

_____

_____

_____

_____

_____

_____

O is for OBEY

But Peter and the apostles replied, "We must obey God rather than any human authority." — Acts 5:29 (NLT)

- Do not obey both God and man;
- God is first because He is your Father;
- Obey God!

I choose to **OBEY** God over man by doing the following:

_____

_____

_____

_____

_____

_____

_____

_____

_____

_____

_____

_____

P is for PRAY

Pray continually. — *1 Thessalonians 5:17 (NIV)*

- Talk to your Father God;
- Talk to God at anytime;
- Reference the Disciples' Prayer (Matthew 6:9-13) as a model.

I **PRAY** during this daily scheduled time frame:

_____

_____

_____

_____

_____

_____

_____

_____

_____

_____

_____

Q is for QUIET

You should clothe yourselves instead with the beauty that come from within, the unfading beauty of a gentle and quiet spirit, which is so precious to God. — 1 Peter 3:4 (NLT)

- Your beauty is from within;
- The Holy Spirit lives within you;
- The Holy Spirit should take over your outward/physical beauty showing of gentleness and quietness.

The gentle and **QUIET** Spirit radiates as I do the following:

R is for RESIST

Resist the devil and he will flee from you. — James 4:7b (NIV)

- Do not give into things that cause you to sin;
- Say "no" to people and acts whose desire is to partake in something contrary to God and His Word;
- During consistent prayer time, ask God to help you not to give in to sin although it's part of our nature to do so.

I **RESIST** the devil by doing the following:

_____

_____

_____

_____

_____

_____

_____

_____

_____

_____

S is for SUBMIT

Submit yourselves, then, to God. — *James 4:7a (NIV)*

- Submit to God daily;
- Give everything to God daily;
- Give all of you to God daily.

    I **SUBMIT** myself to God by doing the following:

_____

_____

_____

_____

_____

_____

_____

_____

_____

_____

_____

T is for TRUST

Trust in the Lord with all your heart and lean not on your own understanding. — Proverbs 3:5 (NIV)

- Trust the Lord;
- Trust the Lord in everything;
- The Lord is only one to trust.

*I display my **TRUST** in the Lord by doing the following:*

_____

_____

_____

_____

_____

_____

_____

_____

_____

_____

_____

U is for UNDERSTANDING

A man who lacks judgement derides his neighbor, but a man of understanding hold his tongue. — Proverbs 11:12 (NIV)

- Have understanding means not speaking at all;
- You do not have to speak in response to someone else's words;
- Realize that what you say can either destroy or encourage.

I demonstrate being a person of **UNDERSTANDING** by responding in these ways:

_____

_____

_____

_____

_____

_____

_____

_____

_____

_____

V is for VICTORY

With God we will gain the victory, and he will trample down our enemies. — *Psalm 60: 1-2 (NIV)*

- You are victorious;
- God fights for you when you're still;
- You are to be in relationship with God to gain the victory.

I have **VICTORY** in my:

_____

_____

_____

_____

_____

_____

_____

_____

_____

_____

_____

W is for WISDOM

The fear of the Lord is the beginning of wisdom, all who follow his precepts have good understanding. To him belongs eternal praise. — Psalm 111:10 (NIV)

- You begin to obtain wisdom by fearing the Lord;
- Fear the Lord by doing what His Word states;
- Be wise by understanding and obeying God's Word.

I have **WISDOM** as I do the following:

_____

_____

_____

_____

_____

_____

_____

_____

_____

_____

X is for eXODUS

The Lord himself will fight for you. Just stay calm. — *Exodus 14:14 (NLT)*

- Maintain a positive attitude;
- You will rise and make it;
- Think consistently on encouraging words so they outnumber anything negative.

I will remain calm as in **eXODUS** by doing the following:

_____

_____

_____

_____

_____

_____

_____

_____

_____

_____

_____

_____

Y is for YESTERDAY

Jesus is the same yesterday, today and forever. — *Hebrews 13:8 (NIV)*

- Jesus never changes;
- Jesus is always the same;
- Count on Jesus daily.

Jesus shows me He's the same **YESTERDAY**:

_____

_____

_____

_____

_____

_____

_____

_____

_____

_____

_____

_____

Z is for ZEAL

Never be lacking in zeal, but keep your spiritual fervor,
serving the Lord. — Romans 12:11 (NIV)

- Keep your zeal;
- Serve the Lord;
- Maintain your spiritual fervor.

I keep my **ZEAL** by doing:

_____

_____

_____

_____

_____

_____

_____

_____

_____

_____

_____

_____

About the Author

Mary P. Wells is the Founder & President of *One Word Encourage, LLC*. She shares encouraging words so people continuously speak, wear and live an abundant life. She creates daily posts to motivate her followers to be better in every area of their lives.

As a Breast Cancer Survivor, Mary hosts the annual "Got Treatment, Now Thrive" public event to provide post- treatment advice and support.

Also, Mary volunteers through community service partnerships with *EACH Outreach* and *Our Favorite Things Boutique*. She volunteers in homeless shelters, and serves as a guest speaker at the annual Elizabeth Maddox Breast Cancer Memorial to an audience who supports Awareness.

Mary received her Bachelor of Arts degree in English from The Ohio State University. She is a dedicated mother to her son and continues to live in Cleveland, Ohio, where she was born and raised.